VIAGRA

FOR MEN

The Best Guide that explains the Use of Viagra Pills to Cure
Erectile Dysfunction, Premature Ejaculation, Increase Libido
and for Improved Intimacy

Dr. Shun Joe

TABLE OF CONTENT

i

1

INTRODUCTION

Most people find it difficult to stick with their weight loss plan, which has given their hope for weight loss a daunting routine. There are effective methods for losing weight rapidly and efficiently and keeping it off. If you combine the recipe in this book along with regular exercise, you may also be able to strengthen your immune system accompanied with a rapid weight loss.

The recipe in this book produces weight loss comparable to other diets supervised by a nutrition professional. This book includes easy-to-follow recipes for a variety of wholesome main dishes plus sweet and savory desserts. You won't go hungry even if you're a weight watcher because there are foods on the menu that are high in fiber, low in carbohydrates, high in unsaturated fat (healthy fats), and high in lean protein.

BREAKFAST RECIEPE SAMPLES

1

CINNAMON APPLE OATMEAL

This breakfast contains 312 calories 7grams of protein and 4.7grams of fiber. Because of their high soluble fibre content, oats are excellent for decreasing cholesterol.

Ingredients

These ingredients make for 2 servings

- oats that are quick to cook or traditional (1 cup)
- (2/3 cups) of apple juice concentrate
- (1 1/3 cups) of water
- (1/2 teaspoon) cinnamon
- (1/2 cup) currants or raisins

Directions

1. In a saucepan, mix the oats, water, apple juice concentrate, and cinnamon.
2. Bring to a simmer, then cook for three minutes with a lid on.
3. If using, remove from heat and mix in the raisins or currants. 3 minutes should pass before serving.

Nutrition

Nutritional value Per serving (1 cup)

- *Calories 312 per serving*
- *Total Fat: 2.9 g*
- *Saturated Fat: 0.5 g*
- *Calories from Fat: 8.4%*
- *7 g of protein*
- *66 g of carbohydrate*
- *32.9 g of sugar*
- *4.7 g of fiber*
- *29 mg of Sodium*
- *51 mg of Calcium*
- *2.8 mg of Iron*
- *2.1 mg of Vitamin C*
- *0.3 mg of Vitamin E*

2

SPICED PUMPKIN BREAD

A breakfast, of a moist, delicious bread that is spiced to perfection. A slice of this bread contains 140 calories 3gram of protein and 4gram of fiber. Vitamins A and C are abundant nutrient in pumpkins, which can strengthen the eater's immune system.

Ingredients

The listed ingredients Makes for 12 slices of bread, equivalent to 1 loaf Serving.

- sifted whole-wheat pastry flour (2 cups)
- baking powder (1 tsp.)
- baking soda (1 tsp.)
- (1/4 teaspoon) sea salt
- flaxseed meal (1.5 tablespoons).
- ground cinnamon (1 tsp.)
- ground ginger (1 tsp.)
- Spice for pumpkin pie (1/2 tsp.)
- Your choice of non-dairy milk (1/2 cup) OR rice milk)
- canned pumpkin puree (1 cup plus 2 tbsp.)
- (Half a cup) maple syrup
- brown rice vinegar (1/2 tsp.)
- pure vanilla extract (1 tsp.) (Half a cup) raisins

Directions

1. Grease a 1 1/2-quart loaf pan and preheat the oven to 350 degrees.

2. Whisk the dry ingredients together in a large bowl (flour, baking powder, baking soda, salt, flaxseed meal, cinnamon, ginger, and pumpkin pie spice)
3. Whisk the rice milk, pumpkin puree, maple syrup, vinegar, and vanilla in a separate basin.
4. To combine, fold the wet and dry ingredients together. Add raisins and fold.
5. Fill the loaf pan evenly with the mixture.
6. Bake for an hour (60 minutes), or until the toothpick inserted into the center comes out clean.
7. Cool down. Keep in a container that is covered.

Nutrition

Per serving (1 slice) 140 calories per slice

- *3 grams of protein*
- *Carbohydrate: 32 grams of carbohydrate*
- *Sugar: 13 grams of sugar*
- *Fat: 1 gram*
- *Calories from Fat: 6%*
- *Fiber: 4 grams*
- *203 mg of sodium*

3

TOFU SCRAMBLE

When extra-firm tofu is crumbled, it offers the texture and flavor of scrambled eggs without any additional cholesterol when combined with turmeric. This breakfast contains 108 Calories 10gram of protein and 4.6 grams of fiber per serving.

Tofu is a great source of plant-based protein, and it may even help prevent some cancers!

Ingredients

These ingredients make for 4 Servings

- extra firm tofu (light or low-fat when possible) 14 to 16 ounces
- 1 clove minced garlic, 1/2 cup diced onion, 1/2 cup diced green pepper, and 1/2 cup diced red pepper
- chopped mushrooms (3/4 cup)
- (1/4 teaspoon) of turmeric powder
- cayenne powder (1 teaspoon)
- (3/4 teaspoon) black pepper
- salt (1 teaspoon)

Directions

1. Large saute pan with 1/4 cup (60 milliliters) water added. Add onion dice once it's warmed up.

2. Add minced garlic when the onion starts to become transparent and gives off its aroma. Cook for a further two minutes before adding diced peppers and chopped mushrooms. If the veggies are sticking to the pan, add 1/4 cup (60 milliliters) of water. Vegetables should be cooked for 4 minutes or until soft.
3. With hands, break up the tofu and add it to the pan with the turmeric after thoroughly combining. Cook for another 4-6 minutes, until everything is thoroughly heated through, before adding cumin powder, pepper, and salt.
4. Serve atop a warm corn tortilla or with whole-grain bread.

Nutrition

Nutritional value Per serving

- *Calories: 108*
- *Fat: 4.6 g*
- *Saturated Fat: 0.6 g*
- *Calories from Fat: 36%*
- *Cholesterol: 0 mg*
- *10 grams of Protein*
- *9.2 grams of Carbohydrate*
    - *3.5gram of sugar*
    - *4.2gram of Fibre*
- *594 mg of Sodium*
- *67 mg of Calcium*
- *3.2 mg of Iron*
- *41.6 mg of Vitamin C*
- *0.5 mg of Vitamin E*

4

BREAKFAST POTATOES

The ideal comfort dish for brunch or breakfast is potatoes! They can also be put on top of grits or maize. combine with fruit. Check the label because not all soy sauces are gluten-free. Tamari is often secure. These potatoes meal contains 128 calories, 3.1grams of protein and 4.1gram fiber per serving.

Ingredients

These ingredients make for 4 Servings

- Red or white potatoes,
- washed (2) onion,
- thinly sliced (1) soy sauce (4 teaspoons),
- sweet paprika or chili powder (1/2 teaspoon),
- dried oregano (1/2 teaspoon),
- poblano pepper,
- chopped into thin strips (1) cherry tomatoes, cut (5-8), green onions, sliced (2)

Directions

1. The potatoes should be washed, cut into 1/2-inch cubes, and steamed for 10 minutes or until just soft. Get rid of the heat.

2. In a big nonstick skillet, heat up 1/4 cup (60 milliliters) of water, then add the onion. Cook, frequently stirring, until the water has evaporated, and the onion has started to adhere to the pan. Add another 1/4 cup (60 milliliters) of water while scraping the pan, then simmer until the onion starts to stick once more. Continue doing this until the onion is fragrant and golden brown. It will take around 15 minutes to complete this.
3. Sprinkle the soy sauce, dry oregano, and sweet paprika over the potatoes and thinly sliced poblano pepper (or chili powder, if preferred). Cook, using a spatula to carefully toss, until the potatoes are thoroughly browned.
4. If desired, top with the sliced green onions and cherry tomatoes.

Nutrition

Nutritional value Per serving (i.e., a quarter of the recipe),
- *128 calories*
- *Saturated Fat: 0.1 g Fat: 0.2 g*
- *1.7 percent of calories come from fat.*
- *0 mg of cholesterol*
- *3.1 g of protein*
- *29.9 g of carbohydrates.*
- *Sucrose: 2.7 g*

- *4.1 g of fiber*
- *Salt: 309 mg*
- *39 mg. of calcium*
- *: 2.7 mg iron*
- *19.5 milligrams of vitamin C*
- *89 mcg Beta-Carotene*
- *0.2 milligrams of vitamin E*

5

Tofu Paneer Bhurji

Serve this tofu scramble in an Indian style wrap or tortilla of your choice, along with rice and Indian flatbread. A portion of these dish contains 101 Calories, 9.5 grams of Protein and 2.1 grams of Fiber.

Ingredients

These ingredients make 4 Servings

- cumin seeds (1 teaspoon)
- Medium onion,
- minced finely (1) Garlic,
- minced (1 clove) Green chiles,
- seeded and minced (1-4) Fresh ginger,
- peeled and minced (1/2-inch piece) Tomatoes,
- minced (2) Turmeric (1/4 tsp.) Garam masala (1 tsp.) Salt (to taste)
- 1 14–16-ounce container of crumbled firm or extra-firm tofu, 3 teaspoons of cashew paste, and 1/4 cup of finely chopped fresh cilantro for garnish)

Directions

1. Add cumin seeds to a big pan and heat it up on medium.
2. Add the onion, garlic, green chilies, and ginger when they begin to splutter.
3. Add the tomatoes, turmeric, curry powder, and salt when the mixture starts to turn brown.

4. Add the tofu and cashew paste, if using, when the tomatoes start to break down. If using, garnish with cilantro.
5. The onion, garlic, chiles, and ginger can all be combined in a food processor to create a paste rather than being minced and finely chopped. This can speed up the cooking process while maintaining excellent flavor.

Nutrition

Nutritional value Per serving (i.e., a quarter of recipe)

- *Calories: 101*
- *Fat: 4.5 g*
- *Saturated Fat: 0.9 g*
- *Calories from Fat: 37.1%*
- *Cholesterol: 0 mg*
- *Protein: 9.5 g*
- *Carbohydrates: 8.6 g*
- *Sugar: 3.4 g*
- *Fiber: 2.1 g*
- *Sodium: 420 mg*
- *Calcium: 222 mg*
- *Iron: 2.7 mg*
- *Vitamin C: 36 mg*
- *Beta Carotene: 237 mcg*
- *Vitamin E: 0.5 mg*

6

SWEET POTATO TOASTS

Sweet potatoes, which are tasty and filling, can elevate regular toast. For an extra flavorful boost, feel free to add a lot more pepper and more lemon juice! Choose your favorite fruit to round out this dinner.

If you are on a gluten-free diet, make sure you get a loaf of bread without gluten.

This meal contains 329 Calories, 11.9 grams of Protein, and   9.8 gram of Fiber per serving.

Ingredients

These ingredients make for 2 Servings

- grain-sprouting bread (2 slices)
- Peeled and mashed sweet potatoes (see Note): 1/2 cup
- (1/2–1 teaspoon) lemon juice
- table salt (1-2 pinches)
- freshly ground pepper (to taste)
- avocado cubes or a spoonful of thinly chopped black olives (2 tbsp.)

Directions

1. Toast the bread.
2. Remove the sweet potato's peel and mash it in a small bowl with 2 1/2 teaspoons (12.5 milliliters) of lemon juice, a dash of salt, and a grind of black pepper (if using).
3. Between each piece of toast, divide the mashed sweet potato, then top with 2 tablespoons (30 milliliters) of diced avocado or, if you'd like, sliced black olives. Serve!

Note: Sweet potatoes can be baked in advance. Put entire sweet potatoes on a parchment-lined baking sheet. Bake for 40 to 60 minutes, or until very soft, at 450 F (232 C). (The length of time required to cook a sweet potato depends on its size.) Store in the freezer for a few months or the refrigerator for up to 6 days before using.

Nutrition

Nutritional value Per serving

- *329 calories*
- *Fat: 5.6 g*
- *0.9 g of saturated fat; 14.7 percent of calories from fat*
- *0 mg of cholesterol*
- *11.9 g of protein*
- *59.1 g of carbohydrates.*

- *11.5 g of sugar*
- *9.8 g of fiber*
- *Salt: 455 mg*
- *168 mg of calcium*
- *: 2.7 mg iron*
- *28.6 mg of vitamin C*
- *mcg of beta-carotene: 14,720*
- *3.1 milligrams of vitamin E*

7

TOFU ZUCCHINI BREAKFAST SCRAMBLE

This tasty breakfast scramble comes together quickly. Serve it over toasted French bread, warm tortillas, or English muffins. This meal contains 70 Calories, 2.6 grams of Protein, and 2.3 grams Fiber per serving.

Ingredients

These ingredients make for 4 Servings

- Water (1/2 cup) diced onion (1) minced garlic (2 cloves)
- finely sliced medium zucchini (2) and diced firm tofu (1/2 pound).
- chili flakes (1 tsp.)
- sodium-reduced soy sauce (1 tbsp.)
- (Half a cup) salsa
- warm tortillas, English muffins, or a taste of French bread (for serving)

Directions

1. In a sizable nonstick skillet, warm 1/2 cup of water.
2. Add the onion and garlic. Cook for about 5 minutes, stirring often over high heat, until tender.
3. Add the tofu, zucchini, and chili powder. Reduce the heat, cook the zucchini for about 5 minutes, stirring often. If additional water is required, add it sparingly to avoid sticking.
4. Add soy sauce and mix.
5. If using, add salsa on top. Serve with toasted French bread, warm tortillas, or English muffins.

Nutrition

Nutritional value Per 1-cup serving

- *70 calories*
- *Fat: 2.6 g*
- *0.5 g of saturated fat; 33.1 percent of calories from fat*
- *0 mg of cholesterol*
    - *g of protein*
    - *g of carbohydrates*
- *Sucrose: 2.9 g*
- *2.3 g of fiber*
- *Salt: 150 mg*
- *136 milligrams of calcium*
- *1.5 mg iron*
- *6.1 milligrams of vitamin C*
- *496 mcg of beta-carotene*
- *0.3 mg of vitamin E*

8

HUEVOS RANCHEROS

A nutritious take on a traditional breakfast dish! A top-notch, fresh salsa will add extra taste! If you are on a gluten-free diet, make sure to choose gluten-free tortillas or toast.

Ingredients

The ingredients make for 4 Servings

- additional firm tofu (8 ounces)
- Cubed Yukon Gold potatoes, one teaspoon of salt, and ground turmeric (2 tsp.)
- (1/2 tsp.) of chili powder
- (Half a cup) salsa
- tortillas or toast pieces (3) fresh cilantro, chopped (3 tbsp.)
- diced Roma tomatoes (1)

Directions

1. Tofu should be broken up in a mixing dish.
2. Potato cooked by steaming for approximately 5 minutes with crumbled tofu cubes.
3. Heat a skillet over medium heat while steaming. For about 3 to 4 minutes, while stirring slowly and softly, add the tofu and salt.
4. Cook for a further minute after adding the potato, turmeric, and chili powder. Add the salsa.
5. Use flour tortillas or toast to wrap the scrambled tofu in equal parts. Add fresh cilantro and tomato on top.

Leftovers: Approximately 3 minutes into heating the scrambled tofu over medium heat, add the salsa. Add the other ingredients and continue to cook for 2 more minutes.

Nutrition

Nutritional value Per serving

- *255 calories*

19

- *Calories from fat: 3.6 g Saturated fat: 0.5 g 12 percent of people are fat.*
- *0 mg of cholesterol*
- *12.4 g of protein*
- *47.5 g of carbohydrates.*
- *Sucrose: 3.8 g*
- *8.4 g of fiber*
- *Salt: 608 mg*
- *Iron: 4.6 mg Calcium: 108 mg*
- *12.6 milligrams of vitamin C*
- *340 mcg of beta-carotene*
- *1.1 milligrams of vitamin E*

LUNCH RECIPE SAMPLES

9

POROTOS GRANADOS

Traditional versions of this dish are made with fresh cranberry beans. But You can also use cannellini beans if you don't have the freshly cranberry beans. When you pour the broth into the pot, if you have access to freshly cranberry beans, add them. Otherwise, you may use cannellini beans. The expected calories gained from per serving of this meal is 404 Calories and 22 grams, 20 grams of protein and fiber respectively.

Ingredients

These ingredients Makes 4 Servings

1. One onion, two garlic cloves, two carrots, two ears of corn, one bunch of fresh basil, one-fourth of a teaspoon of paprika.
2. sparse oregano (1 tsp)
3. Cannellini or Great Northern beans (4 cups)
4. a single butternut squash, vegetable stock (2 cups)

Directions

1. A big skillet should be heated to a medium. 60 ml) of water or broth should be added. Add 1 cup of chopped onion and 1 clove of minced garlic, and boil for 4 minutes, or until the onion is soft and translucent.
2. Cook for 2 minutes or until the corn is soft after adding 1/3 cup of sliced carrots, corn with the kernels removed, and 2 teaspoons of chopped basil. Oregano and sweet paprika (pimentón dulce) should be mixed together. 2 1/2 cups of cubed butternut squash and broth should be added. Turn down the heat to low, cover, and simmer for about 15 minutes, or until the

butternut squash is soft but firm. Pour in the previously rinsed and drained beans during the final five minutes of cooking. Use salt and pepper to taste to season. Serve.

Nutrition

The complete nutritional value Per Serving:

- *404 calories*
- *Fat total: 2 g*
- *0.3 g of saturated fat*
- *Fat calories: 4% of total calories*
- *0 mg of cholesterol*
- *22 g of protein*
- *83 g of carbohydrates*
- *9.3 g of sugar*
- *20 g of fiber*
- *Salt: 94 mg*
- *273 mg calcium*
- *9 mg. iron*
- *38 mg of vitamin C*
- *mcg of beta-carotene: 15,186*
- *5 mg of vitamin E*

10

VEGGIE EMPANADAS

These vegetarian empanadas are ideal for on-the-go consumption. You'll be left wanting more as lentils and a ton of spices take center stage! Serve with a sofrito or chimichurri that is oil-free. The expected calories from this meal 167 Calories, 7 grams of Protein and 3.8 grams of Fiber per serving.

Ingredients

These ingredients Makes for 16 Servings

1. (3 1/3 cups) of all-purpose flour
2. 1 tsp. salt, 1 cup of warm water, 3 cups of rinsed and sorted brown lentils, and 1 1/3 cups of silken tofu
3. chopped yellow onion (for lentil mix) (1) finely sliced yellow onion; (1/2) bay leaf (for filling) (3/4 cup)
4. minced garlic cloves (2) hot or smoked paprika (2 teaspoons), and sweet paprika (1 tsp.)
5. Ground cumin (1 tsp) sliced olives (1/4 cup), green onions (1/4 cup), raisins (1 tbl), vegetable broth (3/4 cup), and aquafaba (liquid from can of chickpeas) (1/4 cup) are the ingredients.

Directions

1. The all-purpose flour, salt, and tofu should be combined in a big basin to produce the dough. To incorporate the tofu into the flour mixture, either use a pastry cutter or your hands. With a wooden spoon, gradually pour in the heated water and stir.
2. Create a dough ball and knead the dough for 10 minutes on a lightly dusted surface, or until it is smooth and elastic. Put in a bowl, cover, and let sit for an hour.
3. Put the lentils in a small saucepot and add water to cover them to create lentils. Bring to a simmer after adding the bay leaf and half an onion. Lentils should be cooked for 15 minutes

or until just barely soft. Take lentils from the fire and drain them. Put down and let it cool.

4. To make lentils resemble crumbled meat, pulse them in a food processor or mash them with a fork.

5. 1/4 cup of water and a big sauté pan on medium-low heat. When the onion is soft and translucent, add it and cook for an additional 6-7 minutes. Cook for two more minutes after adding the garlic.

6. Cumin, hot and sweet paprika, and lentils should all be added. To mingle, blend. Add the broth and boil for a while. Add green onions, raisins, and olives. Once almost all the liquid has evaporated, continue boiling. according to taste.

7. Set the oven to 350 degrees. Roll out the dough to a thickness of 1/4 inch on a surface dusted with flour. Cut the dough into circles using a big bowl or cookie cutter. Until you have 16 circles, gather any extra dough, roll it into a ball, and repeat the process.

8. One and a half tablespoons of the filling should go in the center of the dough circle. The edges can either be decoratively sealed, as the Argentinians do, or folded over to surround the contents. aquafaba on your brushes.

9. Bake for 35 to 40 minutes, or until the bottoms are golden brown, on a sheet tray covered with parchment paper. Turn the broiler to low while turning the oven off. The empanadas' tops will become brown as a result. Empanades should be broiled for 5 minutes.

Nutrition

The complete nutritional value Per serving:

- *167 calories*
- *Calories from fat: 1.1 g Fat: 0.1 g Saturated fat: 0.1 g Fat: 5%*
- *0 mg of cholesterol*
- *7 g of protein*
- *31 g of carbohydrates*
- *1.9 g of sugar*
- *3.8 g of fiber*
- *Salt: 216 mg*
- *23 mg of calcium*
- *fer: 3 mg*
- *Nutritional C: 1.5 mg*
- *176 mcg of beta-carotene*
- *0.2 milligrams of vitamin E*

11

MEXICAN NOODLE SOUP

In central Mexico, fideo soup is a common dish cooked with tart tomato base and golden-brown noodles. But try experimenting with various peppers, spices, and other ingredients to create the version of this traditional dish that best suits your tastes!

Ingredients

These ingredients Makes for 4 Servings

- (Or thin spaghetti, cut into 1-inch pieces) Fideo noodles (8 ounces)
- tomatoes, diced (one can), white onion, chopped (half), peeled garlic cloves, two chipotle peppers in adobo, and one dry oregano (1 tsp.)
- 1 1/4 cups of chopped zucchini in vegetable broth (2 cups)
- Silken tofu (4 ounces), lemon juice (1/2 tablespoon), garlic clove (1/2), unsweetened almond milk (1 tablespoon), nutritional yeast (1 tsp.)
- Pepper and salt (to taste)
- (1/4 cup) of chopped cilantro)

Directions

1. To make the tomato broth, place the diced tomatoes, chipotle pepper, onion, garlic, and 1 cup of broth into a food processor and process until smooth. Set aside.
2. Set a large pot to medium heat. Add noodles and dry toast them until golden brown. Add tomato broth and let simmer, stirring constantly, until the tomato broth turns a deep red color about 2 minutes. Add zucchini, oregano, and remaining 1/2 cup of broth.
3. Turn heat to low and continue simmering and stirring until the noodles and zucchini are tender, about 10 to 12 minutes. Season to taste.
4. While the noodles are simmering, place the tofu, lemon juice, garlic, and nutritional yeast in the blender and process until smooth. Season to taste.

5. If there is too much liquid in your noodles, let them sit for 5 minutes and let the pasta absorb the excess moisture.
6. Place noodles on a serving dish and drizzle the tofu crema on the noodles and sprinkle with chopped cilantro.

Nutrition

Complete nutritional value Per serving:

- *328 calories*
- *Fat: 3.6 g*
- *0.6 g of saturated fat*
- *Energy from 9 percent of people are fat.*
- *0 mg of cholesterol*
- *15 g of protein*
- *58 g of carbohydrates*
- *Sucrose: 6 g*
- *Glucose: 5.8 g*
- *Salt: 393 mg*
- *98 milligrams of calcium*
- *: 3.6 mg iron*
- *21 mg of vitamin C*
- *650 mcg of beta-carotene*
- *0.1 mg of vitamin E*

12

EASY BEAN SALAD

This classic bean salad comes together quickly and keeps well. For more fiber-rich whole grains, serve it with a tortilla, more corn, brown rice, or quinoa. Additionally, you might serve it on a bed of leafy greens. Beans leftover from the week should be saved!

Beans are a good source of fiber and protein that can improve digestion and decrease cholesterol.

Ingredients

These ingredients Makes for 4 Servings

1. cooked or canned kidney beans, rinsed and drained (1 1/2 cups)
2. cooked or canned pinto beans, rinsed and drained (1 1/2 cups)
3. cooked or canned black-eyed peas, rinsed and drained (1 1/2 cups)
4. frozen lima beans, thawed; or cooked or canned lima beans, rinsed and drained (1 10-ounce package; or 1 1/2 cups)
5. frozen corn, thawed, or cooked fresh corn, chilled (1 cup)
6. large red bell pepper, diced (1)
7. medium red onion, diced (1/2)
8. low-fat or fat-free Italian salad dressing (1/2 cup)
9. salt (1/2-1 tsp.) ground black pepper (1 tsp.)

Directions

If canned, rinse and drain the beans and/or corn. Beans and corn from a can work as well. Bell pepper and onion should be diced. In a big bowl, mix everything together and gently toss. at room temperature or chilly. Leftover Easy Bean Salad keeps for up to 3 days in the refrigerator when kept in a closed container.

Nutrition

The complete nutritional value Per serving:

- *191 calories*
- *Saturated fat: 0.3 g of the 1.4 g of fat*
- *Energy from 6.3% of total is fat.*

- *0 mg of cholesterol*
- *10.4 g of protein*
- *36.2 g of carbohydrates.*
- *7.3 g of sugar*
- *8.3 g of fiber*
- *1146 mg of sodium*
- *72 mg of calcium*
- *: 2.7 mg iron*
- *58.5 mg of vitamin C*
- *849 mcg of beta-carotene*
- *1.3 milligrams of vitamin E*

13

BROCCOLI BURRITOS

These burritos are flavorful thanks to the optional tahini and salsa!

Calcium and vitamin K, which maintain bone health, are abundant in broccoli.

The tortilla is not gluten-free if it is manufactured from wheat, rye, or other grains.

Ingredients
These ingredients make for 4 Servings

1. (2) Garbanzo beans and broccoli stems (1 15-ounce can)

2. (1/2 cup) roasted red peppers

3. tahini (2 tbsp.)

4. citrus juice (3 tbsp.)

5. salsa, four wheat tortillas (6 tbsp. or more to taste)

Directions

1. Broccoli florets should be cut or broken. Slice peeled stalks into 1/2-inch (1.3 cm) rounds. It takes around 5 minutes to steam broccoli over boiling water until it's just about tender.

2. Put cooked chickpeas (dry and rinse if canned), 1/2 cup (78 grams) of chopped roasted red pepper, tahini (if using), and 4 tablespoons (60 milliliters) of fresh lemon juice in a food processor. About two minutes, or until perfectly smooth.

3. Spread a tortilla with about 1/4 of the chickpea mixture, then put it in a sizable, hot skillet. About 2 minutes of heating will make the tortilla warm and pliable. Spread salsa over the cooked broccoli in the center, then arrange the broccoli in a line. Wrap the tortilla around the filling, then turn off the heat. the remaining tortillas and repeat and serve warm.

Nutrition

The complete nutritional value Per serving

- *305 calories*
- *Sugar: 7.7 g Protein: 14.7 g Carbohydrate: 57.6 g*
- *Fat total: 4.1 g*
- *0.4 g of saturated fat*
- *11.4 % of calories from fat*
- *11 g of fiber*
- *Calcium: 114 mg Sodium: 725 mg*
- *: 3.1 mg iron*
- *106.6 mg of vitamin C*
- *664 mcg of beta-carotene*
- *2.2 milligrams of vitamin E*

14

SUBJI

Subji is so yummy with brown rice or when served with whole wheat chapati.

Ingredients

These ingredients make for 4 Servings

1. Red amaranth leaves (2 1/2 cups), fenugreek (methi) leaves (1 cup), and dill leaves or fresh dill (1/2 cup) should all be cut coarsely.

2. Medium red onion, finely chopped; one entire red Chile, broken into two pieces; or 1/2 to 1 teaspoon dried chili flakes; three to four urad dal (black gram dal); one tablespoon mustard seeds; half a teaspoon curry leaves; and eight to ten cloves of garlic, finely minced (4-5 cloves)
3. Red chili powder or 1/4 teaspoon cayenne pepper (1/2 teaspoon), turmeric powder (1/2 teaspoon), crushed or powdered roasted peanuts (2-4 tablespoons), tamarind soaked in 1 tablespoon of water, or 1/2 teaspoon tamarind paste (1 tsp.)

Directions

1. Dry toast mustard seeds over medium heat in a pan.
2. Add urad dal and stir when they begin to sputter. Roast till golden.
3. For a few seconds, add the garlic, curry leaves, and whole red chili.
4. When the onion is transparent, add it and continue to cook it while adding a tablespoon of water if it begins to burn.
5. Stir in the red chili powder and turmeric powder for a minute or two.
6. Greens should be added and sautéed for 2–3 minutes.
7. Greens should be fully cooked after 5 to 10 minutes of cooking in a covered skillet.
8. Mix well before adding the peanut powder and tamarind pulp.
9. The greens are prepared for serving after one more minute of cooking.

Nutrition

The complete nutritional value Per serving (1/4 of recipe)

- *74 calories*
- *Fat: 3 g*
- *0.5 g of saturated fat*
- *Energy from 31 percent is fat*
- *0 mg of cholesterol*
- *4 g of protein*
- *10 g of carbohydrates*
- *Sucrose: 3 g*
- *3 g of fiber*
- *Salt: 31 mg*
- *74 mg of calcium*
- *fer: 2 mg*
- *84 mg of vitamin C*
- *776 mcg of beta-carotene*
- *1 mg of vitamin E*
- *392 milligrams of potassium*

15

Zucchini Noodles with Dried Tomato Sauce

This lunchtime dish is delicious and straightforward. To add more lasting power to this recipe, drain and rinse a can of white beans. Warm whole grain bread should be served alongside.

Ingredients

These ingredients Makes for 2 Serving

- (2) Fresh basil leaves, two zucchini (to taste)
- Garlic (1/2 clove), tomato, diced (2 tablespoons)
- 1/2 cup of sun-dried tomatoes
- vinegar of balsam (1 tbsp.)
- new thyme (1 tsp.)
- (1/4 teaspoon) freshly ground black pepper
- water as necessary)

Directions

1. Making the sauce: The fresh tomato should be chopped before being added to a blender with a

small garlic clove. After blending for 30 seconds, add the crushed pepper, ground thyme leaves, balsamic vinegar, and the equivalent of a 1/2 cup (28 grams) of sun-dried tomatoes. Depending on how thick or thin you want the sauce to be, add water as necessary.

2. Apply a vegetable peeler to the zucchini and slice it lengthwise. Don't throw away the peel. It is a component of zucchini pasta!

3. Add the sauce to the zucchini, then top with basil (whole or thinly chopped, to taste), pine nuts, and cheese.

Nutrition

The complete nutritional diet Per serving

- *154 calories*
- *8 g of protein*
- *29 g of carbohydrates*
- *Sucrose: 17 g*
- *3 g total fat*
- *Fat calories: 16% of total calories*
- *8 g of fiber*
- *Salt: 71 mg*

16

BLUE CORN CHIP SALAD

Both the eyes and the mount will be delighted by blue corn chips.

Verify that no wheat has been added to the list of ingredients for the blue corn chips

Ingredients

These ingredient makes for 2 Servings

1. Blue corn chips that have been cooked; alternatively, other colored corn chips (4 cups) cooked, rinsed, 16-ounce can of black beans; small head of red leaf lettuce torn into bite-sized pieces; salsa (1 cup)
2. Roasted red peppers, chopped into 2" long by 1/2" thick strips; three diced Roma tomatoes; one tablespoon of green pumpkin seeds.

Directions

1. First, put the corn chips on the plates. You may use any baked corn chips, but blue adds a little color!
2. The lettuce, cut into bite-sized slices, should then be added.

3. After that, add roasted red peppers that have been cut into strips that are 2 inches long and 1/2 inch thick.
4. Add the salsa, tomatoes, and beans as a garnish.
5. Options: If you decide to use green pumpkin seeds, add them last to the salad.
6. Fundamental Ideas: Baked corn chips make fantastic croutons. They are the ideal replacement for the bread-like, typically fried and oil-filled varieties.

Nutrition

The complete nutritional diet Per serving

- *239 calories*
- *10 g of protein*
- *39 g of carbohydrates*
- *16 g of sugar*
- *Fat total: 2 g*
- *9% of calories come from fat*
- *15 g of fiber*
- *Salt: 340 mg*

17

WARM CHILI MAC

This delectable chili and pasta dish will appeal to kids of all ages.

Beans, which are wholesome and high in fiber and protein, are included in this hearty chili.

Ingredients

These ingredients Makes for 10 Servings

1. noodles that are not wet (8 ounces)
2. (1/2 cup) of water
3. Small red or green pepper, diced; 1 minced (3 cloves) onion; 1 vegetarian ground beef alternative; or 4 veggie burgers, thawed (if necessary), chopped (1 8-ounce package)
4. kidney beans, undrained (1 15 ounce can), undrained corn, and crushed tomatoes (1 28 ounce can) (1 15-ounce can)
5. cumin and two tablespoons of chili powder (1 tsp.)

Directions

1. Macaroni should be prepared as directed on the packaging. Rinse, drain, and put away.
2. In a big pot, heat the water. Add the onion and garlic. About 5 minutes of cooking will soften the onion.
3. Add bell pepper and chopped vegetarian burgers or a vegetarian ground beef alternative. Add the

tomatoes, liquid from the beans and corn, cumin, chili powder, and their respective liquids. For 20 minutes, simmer with the lid on over medium heat while stirring occasionally.

4. After adding cooked pasta, taste for seasoning. If you want your dish to be spicier, add additional chili powder.

Nutrition

The complete nutritional diet Per serving

- *211 calories*
  - o *2.1 g of fat and 0.3 g of saturated fat*
- *8.7% of Calories comes from Fat:*
- *0 mg of cholesterol*
- *12 g of protein*
- *38.3 g of carbohydrates.*
- *Sucrose: 4.7 g*
  - o *5.1g of fiber*
- *Salt: 348 mg*
- *62 mg of calcium*
- *: 3.5 mg iron*
- *23.9 mg of vitamin C*
- *450 mcg of beta-carotene*
- *1.3 milligrams of vitamin E*

18

SOBA NOODLES WITH CHINESE VEGETABLES

This is an Asian-inspired meal brimming with vibrant veggies that have been cooked to a nice texture and served al dente. You can take it cold or hot.

Ingredients

Makes for 4 2-cup Servings

1. Ramen noodles (1 8-ounce package)
2. Medium carrots, peeled, cut into half-moon slices (2) Red bell pepper, cut into strips (1) Sugar snap peas (1 cup) Savoy cabbage, sliced (1 cup), vegetable broth (1/2 cup), small leek, white part only, washed and thinly sliced (1) fresh peeled minced ginger (1 tbsp), garlic, minced (2 cloves), cilantro leaves for garnish (to taste)

Directions

1. Follow the instructions on the package for cooking the noodles. Rinse, drain, and put away.
2. In a wok or large skillet over high heat, warm 1/4 cup stock. Stir-fry the leek for 2 minutes after adding it. Stir-fry the carrots, ginger, and garlic for two minutes.
3. Add the cabbage, bell pepper, and remaining 1/4 cup of stock. Vegetables should be steam-steamed for 3 to 5 minutes, covered. Cook for one minute after adding sugar and soy sauce. To reheat, include the noodles.

4. To serve, place the noodles on a dish and garnish with cilantro.

Nutrition

Per serving (1/4 of recipe)

- *229 calories*
- *1 g fat, 0.2 g of it saturated*
- *Energy from Fat: 3.7 percent*
- *0 mg of cholesterol*
    - *9.8g of protein*
- *49.4 g of carbohydrates.*
- *Sucrose: 6.9 g*
    - *6.4g of fiber*
- *Salt: 411 mg*
- *Iron: 2.5 mg Calcium: 53 mg*
- *60.9 mg of vitamin C*
- *2,953 mcg of beta-carotene*
- *1.3 milligrams of vitamin E*

19

ZIPPY YAMS AND BOK CHOY

This dish has a delicious zip thanks to the chili paste, lemon, and garlic, and it's a cheap way to eat nutrient-rich vegetables like yams and bok choy. Bok choy is a fantastic source of calcium and folate and is included in this dish. Even without the vegetarian Worcestershire sauce, the dish will still be flavorful if you do without it.

Ingredients

These ingredient Makes for 4 Servings

1. tiny yams, diced into bite-sized pieces (2) quartered and sliced onion (1) minced garlic (2 cloves)
2. Worcestershire sauce made without meat (1 tbsp.)
3. (1/2 teaspoon) Thai chili paste
4. Lemon (1/2), two small heads of bok choy, thinly sliced

Directions

1. Place the yams in a large skillet with just enough water to cover them. When yams are mushy when probed with a fork, boil them for 5 to 10 minutes in a covered skillet.
2. Add the onion and garlic, then cook the mixture until roughly half the water has evaporated.
3. Bok choy, chile paste, and vegetarian Worcestershire sauce should be added. Bok choy is cooked when it is tender.
4. Serve the mixture after adding lemon juice.

Nutrition

The complete nutritional diet Per serving (1/4 of recipe)

- *88 calories*
- *Fat: 0.6 g*
- *calories from fat: 6.3 percent Saturated Fat: 0.1 g*
- *0 mg of cholesterol*
- *6 g of protein*
- *17.5 g of carbohydrates.*
- *Sucrose: 7.4 g*
- *4.8 g of fiber*
- *Salt: 172 mg*
- *Iron: 3.8 mg Calcium: 315 mg*
- *91 mg of vitamin C*
- *12,247 mcg of beta-carotene*
- *0.6 mg of vitamin E*

DINNER RECIPE SAMPLES

20

MUSHROOM SANCOCHO

Use small orange or red sweet bell peppers instead of sweet chili peppers if you can't find them. You can omit taro if you can't locate it.

Ingredients

This ingredient Makes for 6 Servings

1. 25 button mushrooms, 1 lb of shiitake mushrooms, 1 onion, 2 green bell peppers, 3 Roma tomatoes, and 4 vegetable broth (4 cups)
2. (1/4 bunch) of cilantro

3. yuca (1 1/2) ears of corn (2) taro; green plantain (1) yellow plantain (1) sweet potato (1) butternut squash (1) chayote squash (1)

Directions

1. A big pot or Dutch oven should be heated to medium-high. Button and shiitake or oyster mushrooms are combined with 1/4 cup (60 ml) of water (approximately 1 lb or 453 g). Sauté mushrooms for 4 minutes, or until they begin to brown and adhere to the bottom of the pot. Pour a small amount of water into the saucepan to deglaze it and remove the delicious brown mushrooms from the bottom. The sancocho will acquire a rich mushroom taste as a result.

2. Stir in 3/4 cup of chopped bell pepper, minced garlic, onion, and sweet chili pepper after lowering heat to low-medium. Cook for 3 minutes, or until the onion is transparent and tender. Cook for an additional 2 minutes, or until the tomatoes begin to break down, after stirring in the chopped tomatoes. Pour in the broth, three cilantro sprigs, green and yellow plantains that have been peeled and sliced, one cup of diced sweet potato, one and a half cups of diced butternut squash, one cup of diced chayote, one and a half cups of diced yuca, one cup of diced taro, and one cup of diced corn. If more broth is required, pour it over the vegetables. Cook for

30 minutes, or until the yuca is soft, after bringing to a simmer. according to taste.

Nutrition

The complete nutritional diet Per Serving

- *198 calories*
- *8 g of total fat.*
- *1.4 g of saturated fat*
- *Energy from 36 percent are fat*
- *0 mg of cholesterol*
- *8 g of protein*
- *27 g of carbohydrates*
- *Sucrose: 5 g*
- *3 g of fiber*
- *Salt: 126 mg*
- *106 milligrams of calcium*
- *: 1.8 mg iron*
- *5 mg of vitamin C*
- *98 mcg Beta-Carotene*
- *0.4 milligrams of vitamin E*

21

Zucchini Noodles With Garlic-Roasted Tomato Sauce

These flavorful, gluten-free zucchini and squash noodles are a wonderful substitute for pasta.

The Physicians Committee's Universal Meals program, which adheres to a straightforward set of criteria and accommodates a wide variety of dietary preferences, is where this recipe was created. Animal-derived products, gluten-containing grains, and common allergies are not present in this Meal.

Ingredients

These ingredient Makes for 4 Servings

1. Two medium green zucchini squash, two medium yellow squash, two medium shallots,

one tablespoon of minced garlic, and ten cherry tomatoes, cut in half (4 tbsp.)
2. salt (to taste)
3. pepper (to taste)
4. new basil (to taste)

Directions

1. Wash and dry the zucchini and squash first. After that, split the zucchini and squash in half and remove the stems. To create spaghetti-like noodles from the squash and zucchini, use a vegetable spiralizer.
2. Shallots are peeled and cut into tiny circles.
3. A 24-inch skillet with olive oil (if using) should be heated until smoking. If you'd like, you can omit the oil by substituting water for it or by using a nonstick pan. Add shallots, garlic, zucchini noodles, and reduce heat to medium-low.
4. For two minutes, stir with a wooden spoon. including cherry tomatoes Cook while stirring for 5 minutes.
5. Serve hot in a bowl with fresh basil and scallions after seasoning and adding fresh basil.

Nutrition

The complete nutritional value Per serving

- *177 calories*
- *Fat: 14.39 g*
- *2.04 g of saturated fat.*
- *Fat-related calories: 71.44 percent*
- *0 mg of cholesterol*

- o *3.11g of protein*
- *12.22 g of carbohydrates*
  - o *6.64g of sugar*
- *3.85 g of fiber*
- *Salt: 9 mg*
- *79 milligrams of calcium*
- *Metal: 1.39 mg*
- *26.33 mg of vitamin C*
- *916 mcg of beta-carotene*
- *2.45 milligrams of vitamin E*

22

ITALIAN FUSILLI WITH SUN-DRIED TOMATOES AND

ARTICHOKE HEARTS

This meal pairs sun-dried tomatoes and artichokes to perfection. The next day, the flavors are even more striking.

Ingredients

These ingredients will Make for 4 Servings

1. Vegetable broth (1/2 cup) and sun-dried tomatoes
2. 1 minced garlic clove, 1 medium onion, 3 drained and quartered artichoke hearts, 1 (14 ounce) can
3. (1/2 cup) dry white wine and sea salt (to taste)
4. freshly ground pepper (to taste)
5. sliced fresh oregano (2 tsp.)

6. Fusilli pasta, preferably whole wheat, thinly sliced fresh basil, and 1 (10-ounce) bag of loosely packed fusilli.

Directions

1. In a small bowl, place the sun-dried tomatoes and cover with boiling water. Let stand for 10 minutes to soften. Tomatoes are drained and then cut into thin strips. Place aside.
2. Broth is heated at a medium-high temperature. For 3 to 5 minutes, until softened and translucent, add the onion and garlic. Tomatoes, artichoke hearts, wine, salt, and black pepper should all be added. Reduce heat, then simmer for five minutes. Basil and oregano are mixed in.
3. In the meantime, prepare the pasta as directed on the package until it is al dente. Drain. Mix the artichoke mixture with the spaghetti.

Nutrition

The complete nutritional value Per Serving

- *401 calories*
- *14.8 g of protein*
- *76.3 g of carbohydrates, 5.7 g of sugar*
- *Fat total: 2.3 g*
- *Fat-related calories: 4.9 percent*
- *10.6 g of fiber*
- *525 milligrams of sodium*

23

SHIITAKE MISO SOUP

Ingredients

These ingredients Makes 4 Servings

1. Thin spaghetti or Asian noodles (4 ounces)
2. Low-sodium vegetable broth (1 quart), minced garlic, chopped green onions, 8 ounces of sliced shiitake mushrooms, and 1 cup (2 cloves)
3. Miso pastes or low-sodium soy sauce, sliced (2) carrots, and 1 tablespoon of chopped ginger (2-3 tbsp.)
4. sodium-free soy sauce (1 tbsp.)
5. either spinach or minced cabbage (2 cups)
6. Flakes of red pepper or Sriracha (to taste)

Directions

Assemble all ingredients as mentioned above. Noodles should be cooked according to the package instructions until they are al dente. Drain, rinsing with cold water before setting aside.

Ingredients for miso soup

In the meantime, add 1/4 cup of broth to a big pot. When the mushrooms are nearly soft, add them.

Cooking Mushrooms

Green onions, garlic, and ginger are then added. Cook until the green onions are transparent, adding a little water if necessary.

Cooking Mushrooms and Green Onions

Add carrots and remaining broth, stirring. When the carrots are soft, turn down the heat, cover, and simmer. Miso and cooked noodles are combined. After letting the mixture sit for a while, taste it and add additional miso (or soy sauce) if necessary.

Noodles in Pot

Just before serving, mix in the spinach (or cabbage). If desired, add red pepper flakes or sriracha. the rest of the green onions as a garnish.

Nutrition

The complete nutritional value Per serving (1/4 of recipe)

- *162 calories*

- *8.3 g of protein, 35 g of carbohydrates.*
- *Sucrose: 5.4 g*
- *Fat total: 0.8 g*
- *Fat calories: 4% of total calories*
  - *4.3 g of fiber*
- *NaCl: 593 mg*

24

SWEET POTATO PUMPKIN SEED CASSEROLE

Ingredients

These ingredients will Make 10 Servings

1. candy potatoes (3 pounds)
2. maple sugar (1 tbsp.)
3. citrus juice (3 tbsp.)
4. cinnamon powder (1/2 tsp.
5. ginger root powder (1/2 tsp.
6. allspice, ground (1/2 tsp.
7. (1/2 teaspoon) orange zest
8. (1/3 cup) chopped, unsweetened apricots
9. (1/4 cup) chopped raw or roasted pumpkin seeds

10.   green and/or white sections of green onions, thinly cut (3 tbsp.)

Directions

set the oven to 400 degrees. To make the potatoes soft to the touch, prick them with a fork several times and bake them in a baking dish for 50 to 60 minutes.

After removing the potatoes from the oven, give them 10 minutes to cool. Throw away the sweet potato peeling and scoop the flesh into a mixing basin. Use a potato masher to gently mash the potatoes until smooth yet slightly lumpy. Stir the sweet potatoes after adding the syrup, orange juice, cinnamon, ginger, allspice, orange zest, and apricots.

Put the pumpkin seeds on top of the mixture before placing it in a casserole dish or 9 by 13-inch baking dish. the seeds should be brown after 20 minutes of baking.

After taking the dish out of the oven, top with the green onions, cut into slices. Serve right away.

Nutrition

The complete nutritional value Per serving

- *145 calories*
- *Fat total: 1.6 g*
- *Energy From 9 percent of people are fat.*
- *30.6 g of carbohydrates, 3.2 g of protein*
- *0 mg of cholesterol*

- ○ *4.5g of fiber*
- *11,664 mcg of beta-carotene*
- *49 milligrams of calcium*
- *Salt: 76 mg*
- *518 milligrams of potassium*

26

VEGAN APPLE SAUSAGE STUFFING

Guests at parties in the fall and winter will be impressed by this cuisine!

Any vegan sausage will do; Field Roast's Smoked Vegan Apple Sage Sausage is a good choice. Use any unsweetened plant milk you like. The chestnuts can be roasted yourself or you can purchase packaged roasted chestnuts. Walnuts are a good substitute for chestnuts if you can't find them.

Ingredients

These ingredients will Make 6 Servings

1. Large carrot, chopped (1) celery stalks, chopped (2) yellow onion, chopped (1) vegan apple sage sausage, diced (8 ounces) roasted chestnuts, chopped (1/4 cup), sage, chopped (1 tsp.), flax egg (1 tbsp. ground flax seed + 2 1/2 tbsp.

water), French bread, cut into large cubes (1 loaf or 7 cups), soy milk, unsweetened (1 cup), vegetable stock, (1 cup), and half tablespoon of salt

Directions

1. Set the oven to 375°F. Spread out the cubed bread on a sheet pan, toast for about 5 minutes in the oven. Place aside.
2. In a blender or food processor, pulse the carrot, onion, and celery until they are reduced to a fine pulp. Place aside.
3. The vegan sausage is added to a big sauté pan that has been heated to medium. Sausage takes around 5-7 minutes to lightly brown when cooked with constant stirring. Take out of the pan and place aside.
4. Sauté pan with vegetable puree added; turn heat to low; and cook for 7 minutes, or until nearly dry. From the pan, remove, and set aside.
5. Sausage, vegetable puree, bread, chestnuts, and finely chopped sage should all be combined in a big bowl.
6. To make the flax egg, combine 1 tbsp. powdered flaxseed with 2 12 tbsp. water in a medium bowl. Observe for five minutes. Salt, vegetable stock, and soy milk should all be added; whisk well. This

should be poured over the bread mixture, then combined.

7. Mixture should be placed in an 8 by 12-inch baking dish, and it should be baked uncovered for 30 minutes or until the top is golden brown.

Nutrition

The complete nutritional value Per serving

- *247 calories*
- *Fat: 6 g*
- *0.6 g of saturated fat*
- *Energy from 19.6% are fat.*
- *0 mg of cholesterol*
- *16.8 g of protein*
- *34 g of carbohydrates*
- *Sucrose: 6 g*
- *4 g of fiber*
- *1,012 mg of sodium*
- *114 milligrams of calcium*
- *: 7.1 mg iron*
  - *3.9 milligrams of vitamin C*
- *999 mcg of beta-carotene*
- *1.3 milligrams of vitamin E*

27

VEGAN BUTTERNUT SQUASH MAC AND "CHEESE"

This vegan mac and cheese's cheesy flavor come from a combination of nutritional yeast and butternut squash.

Beta-carotene, which is abundant in butternut squash, has immune-boosting properties and may even reduce the risk of developing some cancers.

Ingredients

These ingredients will Make 6 Servings

1. medium (1) butternut squash, soy milk (3 cups)
2. Ground mustard (1 tsp), nutritional yeast (4 tbsp), cornstarch (2 tbsp), and garlic powder (1 tsp.)
3. tobacco paprika (1 tsp.)
4. uncooked, big elbow pasta (1 pound)

5. (1/2 cup) panko breadcrumbs
6. sambal (dash)

Directions

1. Remove the seeds from the butternut squash and cut it into big pieces. To make the butternut squash soft, steam it. An electric pressure cooker can also be used; simply set it on a trivet and add 1 1/2 cups of water. Take advantage of the 10-minute steaming setting.
2. After the butternut squash has been cooked, use a spoon to remove the meat from the skin. Make 2 cups aside for the sauce. Dice the remaining squash and set aside another cup of it.
3. 2 cups of freshly cooked butternut squash, soy milk, corn starch, nutritional yeast, ground mustard, garlic powder, and smoked paprika should all be combined in a blender to form the sauce. up till smooth.
4. Pasta should be cooked as directed on the package in a big pot of salted water that has been brought to a boil.
5. Into a sizable pot that is on low to medium heat, pour the sauce. often stir. Add 1 cup of diced butternut squash and the prepared noodles as soon as the sauce starts to simmer. To mingle, blend.
6. In a 9 by 13-inch baking dish, combine the macaroni and "cheese" with the panko breadcrumbs. For five minutes, place the dish under the low oven broiler to brown the top.

Serve warm. Although there may appear to be a lot of sauce, the pasta will absorb it as it cools.

Nutrition

The complete nutritional value Per serving

- *485 calories*
- *Fat: 6.6 g*
- *0.98 g of saturated fat per 100 calories. Fatty: 11.4%*
- *0 mg of cholesterol*
- *22.4 g of protein*
- *93.9 g of carbohydrates.*
- *Sucrose: 6 g*
- *16.8 g of fiber*
- *Salt: 126 mg*
- *Iron: 6 mg Calcium: 268 mg*
- *25.5 mg of vitamin C*
- *7,679 mcg of beta-carotene*
- *2.8 milligrams of vitamin E*

28

FARRO WITH MISO MUSHROOMS, KALE, AND WALNUTS

According to studies, mushrooms may help prevent minor cognitive impairment! For a tasty, brain-boosting recipe, try Chef Lauren Kretzer's Farro with Miso Mushrooms, Kale, and Walnuts.

Ingredients

These ingredients will Makes 4 Servings

1. Vegetable stock (2 1/2 cups, split)
2. (1/2 tsp.) of salt
3. uncooked pearled farro (1) bay leaf (1 cup)
4. cremini mushrooms, sliced (5 cups)
5. minced kale (6 cups)
6. minced garlic cloves (3), white miso (1 tsp), tamari, and nutritional yeast (1 tbsp.)
7. juice of fresh lemons (1 tbsp.)
8. (1/3 cup) chopped, roasted walnuts
9. black peppercorns, ground (1/8 tsp.)

Directions

1. Add farro, salt, bay leaf, and 2 cups of vegetable stock to a medium pot. Once it comes to a boil, immediately lower the heat to a simmer, cover the pot, and cook for 20 to 25 minutes, or until the farro is cooked and the liquid has been absorbed. With a fork, remove from the heat.
2. While the farro is cooking, heat 1/4 cup of vegetable stock in a large saucepan over medium-high heat. Add the mushrooms and simmer for 5 minutes, or until they are soft, stirring periodically. Remaining 1/4 cup of vegetable stock, kale, garlic, tamari, miso, nutritional yeast, and so on. To blend, stir. Cook for an additional 3–4 minutes over medium heat, or until kale is wilted and tender.
3. To the mushroom and kale combination, add cooked farro. Stir in the lemon juice, black pepper, and the toasted walnuts. Offer warm or room temperature.

Nutrition

The complete nutritional value Per Serving

- *287 calories*
- *Fat: 7 g*
- *0.8 g of saturated fat*
- *Energy from 22 percent are fat*
- *0 mg of cholesterol*
- *13 g of protein*
- *48 g of carbohydrates*

- *Sucrose: 3 g*
- *9 g of fiber*
- *1030 milligrams of sodium*
- *78 milligrams of calcium*
- *fer: 3 mg*
- *14 mg of vitamin C*
- *2435 mcg of beta-carotene*
- *0.8 milligrams of vitamin E*

29

Pasta Fagioli

Ingredients

These ingredients will Make for 8 Servings

1. minimally salty vegetable broth (4 cups)
2. (1) coarsely chopped small onion and (2) tiny garlic cloves (6 cloves)
3. drained Great Northern beans (2 15-ounce cans)
4. tomato juice (1 6-ounce can)
5. smashed tomatoes low in sodium (1 28-ounce can)
6. Farfalle pasta is dry (16 ounces)
7. pepper, black (to taste)
8. chopped fresh basil (2 tablespoons)

Directions

1. In a big pot, heat 2 tablespoons of the vegetable broth. For seven minutes, sauté the onion and garlic.
2. The leftover broth, along with the beans, tomato paste, and crushed tomatoes with their juice,

should all be added to the saucepan. Heat the soup on high until it boils.

3. Pasta should be added, covered, and cooked on medium heat until al dente (about 14 minutes). While cooking, stir the pasta occasionally.
4. Add black pepper according to taste. During the last three minutes of cooking, add the fresh basil.

Nutrition

The complete nutritional value Per serving (1/8 of recipe):

- *393 calories*
- *18 g of protein*
- *76 g of carbohydrates*
- *Sucrose: 7 g*
- *Fat: 2 g*
- *Energy from Fat: 4%*
- *10 g of fiber*
- *518 milligrams of sodium*

30

MINESTRONE

Ingredients

These ingredients will Makes for 4 Servings

1. Potatoes, peeled and diced (2) diced tomatoes (1 28-ounce can), zucchini, chopped (1), onion, chopped (1/2), low-sodium vegetable broth, split (6 cups), garlic, finely chopped (4 cloves), carrots, diced (1 cup), celery, sliced (2 stalks), potatoes, diced (2), and salt and pepper to taste (to taste)
2. drained and washed kidney beans (1 15-ounce can)
3. noodles that are not wet (1 cup)
4. either 1 1/2 cups of frozen lima beans (1/2 cup) or 1 1/2 cups of fresh or frozen chopped spinach.

Directions

1. On low heat, sauté the onion for 4 minutes in 1/4 cup of the veggie broth. 3 minutes later, add the garlic and continue to sauté.
2. Add the remaining vegetable broth together with the carrots, celery, potatoes, and tomatoes. For boiling, turn up the heat to medium-high. Medium-low heat should be used to cook the dish for 20 minutes with the lid on.

3. Then incorporate the zucchini, basil, parsley, black pepper, sea salt, macaroni, lima beans, and basil. To bring the mixture back to a boil, turn up the heat to medium-high.
4. Boil for one minute, then turn down the heat to low and simmer, covered, for a further eight minutes. After adding, boil the spinach for three more minutes.

Nutrition

The complete nutritional value Per serving (1/8 of recipe)

- *203 calories*
- *9 g of protein*
- *41 g of carbohydrates*
- *Sucrose: 7 g*
- *Fat: 1 g*
- *6% of calories come from fat*
- *7 g of fiber*
- *Salt: 396 mg*

31

CRISPY SAGE MASHED SWEET POTATOES

Sweet potatoes, particularly white sweet potatoes make for a creamy texture when cooked and mashed. The sage in this recipe offsets the sweetness of the potatoes.

Sweet potatoes are a great source of vitamin B6, which may help boost brain health.

Ingredients

These ingredients will Makes for 2 Servings

1. cooked sweet potatoes with one teaspoon of salt
2. (1/2 teaspoon) cracked black pepper
3. leaves of sage, cut (6-8)

Directions

Sweet potato should be foil-wrapped. Bake for 45 minutes at 450 F. Sweet potatoes should be mashed with salt and black pepper.

The sage leaves should be lightly toasted until they begin to turn crispy in a small pan over medium heat. Mash the sweet potatoes and top with sage.

Nutrition

The complete nutritional value Per serving

- *112 calories*
- *2 g of protein*
- *26 g of carbohydrates*
- *Sucrose: 5 g*
- *Fat total: 0.1 g*
- *Fat-related calories: 0.8 percent*
- *4 g of fiber*
- *Salt: 342 mg*

The End